The Little Book of Self-Health
Natural Healing for the Uninsured

Dr. Toni Fain
Doctor of Natural Medicine
Licensed Massage Therapist
Certified Clinical Hypnotherapist
Lymph Drainage Technician
Certified Medical Assistant
Certified Master Herbalist
Natural Health and Healing Educator

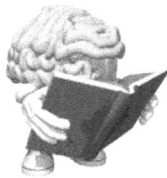

Science tells us that 47% of all healing takes place in the brain.

ISBN 978-0615635828 (paperback)

**The information contained herein
is not intended as medical advice, but
solely as information and education.**
Recommendations of brand-name products do not
reflect sponsorship by any company or other entity.
The author has personal experience with the
products recommended

CONTENTS

1
INTRODUCTION

You need to know this stuff about your body and nutrition, because if you don't take proper care of yourself, who will?

My name is Toni Fain. I am a naturopath, a doctor of natural medicine, and I've been practicing a variety of natural healing techniques for decades. Simply put, I study how the body helps itself heal. I have purchased just about everything there is to purchase from health food stores and worked with just about every ailment. I have researched and helped people with Alzheimer's disease, cancer, stroke, allergies, chronic fatigue syndrome, heart problems, high cholesterol, Candida, colitis, spastic colon, carpal tunnel syndrome, drug addiction, eating disorders, hormone imbalance, insomnia, and menopause symptoms (to name some examples).

Throughout my years helping individuals free themselves from nagging ailments, mental restrictions, and chronic disease, I have found those most willing to try something new or different are those who achieve the greatest results. Some people feel they have nothing left to lose. Others are not satisfied with the traditional methods and approaches available. I intend this book to counter nutritional misinformation that is so rampant these days.

Negative symptoms and chronic complaints arise in those bodies which are in a constant process of breaking down piece-by-piece, organ-by-organ, and cell-by-cell. There are reasons this process manifests itself. I am always amazed that people so easily accept this cell degeneration as part of the aging process.

My passion for health stems from my own personal experiences. I have been healthy most of my life, but my family has encountered a variety of health challenges over the years. It became very clear to me that there was a need to break the "ill health chain." I realized that this was possible. It required nothing more than breaking from past programming, which prevents a person from questioning conventional information and methods, and opening the mind and heart to seek and accept information and methods considered by traditionalists as outside the realm of mainstream thinking. Sometimes good health requires a leap of faith!

Each of the world's cultures has successful methods of dealing with basic approaches to health issues, healing, and disease which we can learn from and borrow. Ayurveda, the "science of life," is one. It has been practiced for 6000 years and is considered the world's most ancient existing medical system. Chinese medicine has been practiced for 6000 years and has "Do no harm" at the core of its philosophy. The Chinese believe that the mind and body are one.

Both disciplines focus on treating the origin of illness rather than merely treating the symptoms. The material I present here follows these philosophies. I am referring to the concepts of working in harmony with the natural healing functions that the body performs every minute of each day, every day throughout one's entire life. Once you discover the baseline foundation that your own body requires, you can build a better health program for yourself. Feed the body its basic daily requirements from natural, organic sources and set yourself free from premature aging, nagging aches, pains, and chronic dysfunction. There are ways to make this happen – from easy to hard, and cheap to expensive.

You can take back control of your life! Stop digesting misinformation. Stop paying doctors, lawyers, and insurance companies to manage your health. If you put as much energy into feeding your body as you do into making sure your insurance covers your prescriptions or your doctor visits, you can be as healthy as you want. Again, the choices are easy versus hard, and cheap versus expensive.

Feel good! Enjoy your life and reach your full potential without the distraction and discomfort of the fatigue, aches, and pains of emerging ailments. Is there anything better than a healthy mind and body? The body, when properly fed the nutrients it requires *can* and *will* heal itself through cell regeneration. You may not want to, or be able to, "eat like a rabbit," common advice on the market today. The information you'll find here will help you balance the eating habits you *do* employ. Follow the simple suggestions outlined in this book and allow yourself at least 90 days, and I promise you will discover the healthy foundation your body requires. You can start living for yourself, today!

DARE TO RISK
To laugh is to risk appearing the fool.
To weep is to risk appearing sentimental.
To reach for another is to risk involvement.
To expose your ideas, your dreams before a crowd, is to risk their loss.
To love is to risk not being loved in return.
To live is to risk dying.
To believe is to risk disappointment.
But risks must be taken because the greatest hazard in life...
is to risk nothing.
The people who risk nothing may avoid suffering and sorrow,
But their self-esteem cannot soar.
They may not learn, feel, change, grow, love or really live life to the fullest.
They are chained by their attitudes.
They become slaves.
They have forfeited their freedom.
ONLY a person who RISKS
is able to experience
REAL FREEDOM.

Author Unknown

2
THE BODY IS MIRACULOUS

The human body is the most magnificent creation on the entire planet! We in the healing arts have discovered that when we employ techniques that will allow it, the body can and will heal itself. If you feed your body at optimum nutritional levels, and clear out all the waste materials, your body is going to regenerate to a healthy state.

Keep in mind that the longer we are on the planet, the more we are exposed to pollutants, chemicals, toxins, and debris that our bodies do not want, cannot use, and cannot rid themselves of. After all, the world is dirtier than it was even 50 years ago. There are more electromagnetic fields that interfere with our natural cellular vibration, assimilation, and elimination.

Every single cell in a body "talks" to other cells. When a toxin or pollutant creates a blockage, it is almost as if one cell is speaking a foreign language which the other cells cannot understand. Therefore, cell communication ceases. If cells cannot communicate, they will not regenerate into a healthy state but will mutate because they have become independent of the others. This independence provides fuel for the mutants to multiply, resulting in disease, imbalance, or illness, and interferes with the body's innate ability to heal itself.

We know that the body consists of approximately 27 trillion cells, of which140 billion die of various natural causes each and every day. The good news is that the body generates 140 billion brand new cells every 24 hours. The oldest cells in our bodies, which are bone cells, are only 7 years old. This means that technically, we grow a new body every 7 years. Skin cells live for only a day or two, yet the skin is the first organ WE NOTICE breaking down even though other parts of the body are in a degenerative process. If the skin starts demonstrating signs of breakdown in just 1 day, can you imagine what is happening to the organs and parts of the body that we can't see?

Here's a question: If our newest muscle cells are only 14 months old, why do our muscles ache after we reach a certain calendar age? Why do our diseases and body disorders return after each new cell cycle? Where is it written that at certain ages we are supposed to accept declining conditions that physically restrict our bodies and lifestyle?

Once upon a time the consensus was that around the age of 40, a person would start wearing eyeglasses and accept diminishing strength. Hands and knees would ache and prevent us from performing simple physical feats. Food would lose its taste. Insomnia, indigestion, heartburn, and puffy feet would become accepted conditions. This acceptance became incorporated into our thinking.

The good news is that good health can be cultivated and practiced. Keep in mind: I think the human body is the most miraculous thing on the planet. After all, we have all heard stories in the news about anorexic adults who weigh 83 pounds, or someone who weighs 1000 pounds – and yet their bodies still function. Not a great way to live, but still living. Pretty miraculous, don't you agree?

We also know that the body is wise and willing to heal itself. Think about how many paper cuts you have experienced over your lifetime. Are they still bleeding? What happened? How did they heal? Did you give instructions to collagen and elastin to repair the cells in the body? Did you write yourself a prescription for healing your paper cut? No. The body, in its wisdom, does this all by itself. A healthy body has been constructing, destructing, and reconstructing cells ever since you were *conceived.*

When a cell replicates or a new cell is born, each can become:

~ More healthy than the original parent cell.

~ Less healthy than the original parent cell.

~ Equally healthy as the original parent cell.

If the cell is equal, your health will maintain its current level. If the cell is less healthy than the original parent cell, then it is breaking down, aging, and becoming less efficient. If, on the other hand, the cell is healthier than the original cell, then you have reversed the aging process and will look and feel better and stronger.

What does it take for a cell to regenerate into a healthier state? It takes fuel. Fuel for a car is gasoline or diesel. Fuel for the human body is food, water, and oxygen. If you are eating the standard American diet, you are probably going to degenerate quickly because that diet is typically loaded with preservatives and chemical additives designed to give your food a longer shelf life. Most of the beverages we drink contain chemistry or preservatives which interfere with the body's access to the nutritional materials it requires for optimum health.

The body has many checks, balances, and fail-safe warnings to signal us when there's a problem already in progress or about to emerge. We need to start paying attention to those signals. Start with the signs that can be observed in the eyes, like dryness, blurred vision, or heaviness or puffiness of the lids. Are the eyes white, yellow, gray, or bloodshot? The less white they are, the more congestion is to blame.

Are your toenails or fingernails riddled with fungus, or dry, brittle, cracked, ridged, ingrown, deformed, or painful? Your skin will be the first to show signs of excess dryness, deeper wrinkling, or skin eruptions that won't heal.

What is the condition of your gums? Are they receding, bleeding, or discolored? The clues are there if we are willing to look and pay attention to them. They are trying to signal that something in our internal body is weakened or stressed. Medical doctors call these signs and signals, "symptoms." The symptoms themselves are not an illness but simply the *language* your body speaks to let you know it is chemically out of harmony.

We need to understand that if we are not healthy we need to take the time to look, really look, at ourselves. If you need to take a picture of yourself to study the outward signs, do it. Additionally, analyze your health by paying attention to your daily routines, especially what you eat and drink. Then examine how these habits affect your health. The following survey is designed to help you recognize the signs of imbalance and potential illness.

This survey will help you become aware of your own health's strengths and challenges. Take it now and then again in 90 days to see what has changed and what areas need more attention.

> **He who rolls up his sleeves seldom loses his shirt.**
> **Anonymous**

3
HEALTH AWARENESS SURVEY

I. General Health

~ Do you have the energy you need to live the life you desire?

~ Do you fall asleep easily, stay asleep, and wake feeling energized?

~ Are you in pain? Identify the areas of your body that are in pain and the frequency of occurrence. It may be helpful to do this over time, making daily notes on a calendar or in a journal.

~ Look at your eyes. Notice if they are clear, blurry, or dry.

~ Examine the whites of your eyes. Are they yellow, gray, or bloodshot?

~ Describe the condition of your skin.

~ Check your tongue. Is it coated? What color is it?

~ Is your hair oily or dry? Brittle or supple?

The Little Book of Self-Health

II. Food

~ What are you eating? Do your eating habits provide the nutritional factors that your body requires to perform and function as it was designed?

~ How many daily servings are you getting of vegetables? Fruits? Proteins? Whole grains? Dairy products?

~ Are you abusing yourself by overindulging or denying what the body requires?

~ How many servings each day do you eat of white flour? Prepackaged foods? Fast foods? White sugar? Junk food?

~ Do you eat raw, fresh fruits and vegetables regularly? Or are they frozen or canned?

~ Is the majority of your diet from organic sources? Or other sources?

~ What oils are listed on the labels of your foods?

~ What oils do you use to cook with?

~ How often do you microwave your food?

~ Do you drink coffee, soda, juice, Red Bull™, or Gatorade™? If yes, with what frequency?

~ How much water do you drink each day?

~ Is your water bottled or from the tap? What is the source of the water?

III. Drugs and Alcohol

~ How much alcohol to you consume?

~ Do you take drugs for recreation? If yes, how fre-
quently? Do these drugs help you cope with the pace
of your life? The stressors?

~ What prescription medications are you using? How
often? For what purpose? For what duration? And do
these drugs help you cope with the pace of your life?
The stressors?

~ What over-the-counter medications are you using?
How often? For what purpose? For what duration? Do
these drugs help you cope with the pace of your life?
The stressors?

IV. Emotional Health & Wellbeing

I have discovered that mental attitude is often overlooked but plays a major role in the quest for a healthier lifestyle. Ask yourself:

~ Do your beliefs or attitudes help or hinder you?

~ Do your physical problems or pains make it hard for
you to find peace and happiness?

~ Are you with a mate? Do you wish to be? Are you
relating to your mate in the way you would like?

~ Do you feel all alone?

~ Are there family and friends readily available to comfort or assist you? If so, is their attitude conducive to your better health?

~ Do you feel your life is nearly over?

~ Have you accomplished what you wanted in life?

~ Are you ready to leave your pain or ailment behind? Or, are you holding onto it because it is attached to an emotional issue? Is there a purpose it is serving in your life? (This is a hard one to answer. Be as honest as you can!)

~ What do you do to be aware of and manage your stress?

~ Do you have quiet time each day?

~ Do you write in a journal?

~ Do you go to a class such as yoga or martial arts?

~ Do you consider yourself religious/spiritual?

~ Do you pray or meditate each day?

V. Breathing

How we breathe is important. There are two kinds of breathing: shallow and deep. Based on the following descriptions, which type of breathing is yours?

~ Shallow: Those who are shallow breathers inhale small amounts of air that only partially fill the lungs to capacity. Shallow breathers have a tendency to be tense, a bit high-strung, and tend to hold onto anguish. As the body is always in want of more air, this keeps the body in a state of anxiety.

~ Deep: Deep breathers inhale larger quantities of air that fill the lungs to a greater capacity, which pushes more air into the bloodstream. Consequently, they tend to be more relaxed and adjust to life's ups-and-downs more readily. Their blood is truly oxygenated.

VI. Lymph System

The lymph system can be thought of as the body's "garbage collector." Its purpose is to protect the body and help it recycle or eliminate what it does not need or want. It is critical that this function remains free of congestion and be allowed to perform its function. When the lymph system is congested or operating sluggishly, the body sends us signals.

Do you have any of the following signs:

~ Congestion?

~ Sinusitis?

~ Bloating?

~ Swelling of glands?

~ Stiffness in the joints?

VII. Elimination

Truly healthy bowels move 20 minutes to 1 hour after EACH meal, at least three times a day if you eat three meals per day.

~ How many bowel movements do you have per day? The fewer the movements, the more the congestion and impacted waste is fermenting and putrefying WITHIN YOUR plumbing.

VIII. Exercise

Do you exercise because you "have to?" Or do you exercise because you are answering your body's urge to move? Do you perceive exercise as a punishment, or a curse?

~ What kinds of exercise do you do? What is the duration? What frequency?

~ Are there activities you love, such as dancing, bicycling, or skiing? How often do you do them?

~ How many hours a day are you sedentary?

~ Do you avoid moving? If yes, why?

Look for any of your answers to this survey that don't stack up the way you want them to. The more you become aware, the more you will recognize the improvements that will result when you follow the suggestions in this book. It may be good to repeat this survey every 90 days to help heighten your awareness and notice changes that are subtle. This will also help you determine if it is time to increase or decrease your nutrient intake.

Now that you are aware, it will be up to you to help yourself heal. Keep an open mind and investigate all the possibilities, theories, and opinions. 100% of the information does not fit 100% of the people 100% of the time.

In addition to mainstream Western medicine and standard doctors, we have Ayurvedic and Chinese medicine practitioners available to us. We have beneficial medicinal herbs from the Amazon and all over the world, and there is medicine in the ocean. Do yourself a favor: Visit a practitioner of Chinese or Ayurvedic medicine. Ask questions and explore all the possibilities. It is your health. It is your body. It is your life. The condition of your mind, spirit, and body are in your hands. With a little work you can get yourself moving in the direction of good health.

There is an answer: Concentrate on nutrition and on removing toxins and blockages from your body. Focus on what you CAN do, then do it.

Read on to discover ways to improve your health.

> **Whoever has control over your health has control over your life. Make sure that person is you!**

4
RESOURCES & TOOLS

D o yourself a favor and go to a health food store or vitamin shop and check their book selection. There are three books I consider "must-haves" in a holistic library.

The first is "Healthy Healing, A Guide to Self-Healing for Everyone" by Linda Rector Page, a naturopath who has written several books, all good. "Healthy Healing" is in its twelfth edition.

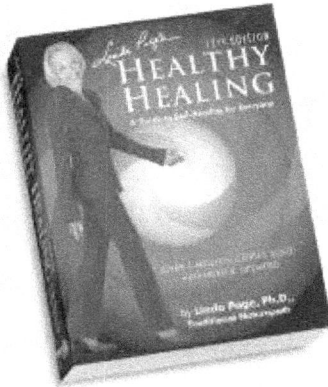

This is the most-used resource book, found in every health food store and worth having as a home reference for any and all symptoms and illnesses your family may encounter.

Another (shown following) is "Prescription for Nutritional Healing: A Practical A-Z Reference for Drug-

Free Remedies Using Vitamins, Minerals, Herbs and Food Supplements," by James and Phyllis Balch.

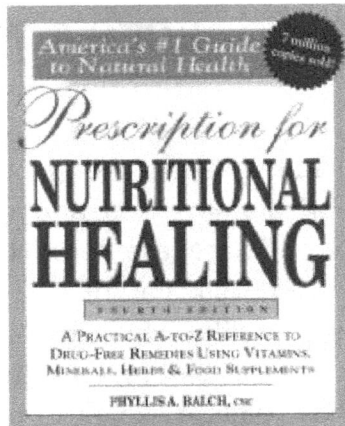

One of the most reliable resource books, loaded with information on specific health challenges and general health and healing information. Worth every penny.

Though these two books seem similar, there are differences. I own both so I can compare and contrast the symptoms I am researching. Having multiple resources helps me make better decisions when following directions for products the authors recommend. In both books you can look up specific symptoms to find a section addressing the ailment along with a list of recommended actions to take. If, for example, they both recommend vitamin C, but only one recommends vitamin E, then I know that C is a safe bet and a good place to start. This will provide me an effective starting point.

The book I recommend on the subject of acid versus alkalinity accompanies a pH testing kit published by Deborah Page Johnson, BFA.

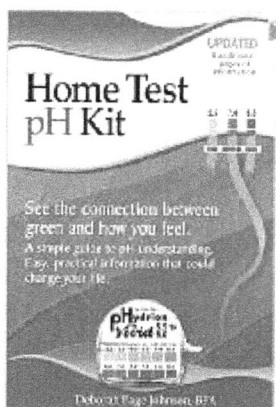

It is sold at health food stores, not bookstores (you might look for it online), and comes with testing paper. You will find it easy to read and follow, and packed with important information.

Muscle Testing

Applied kinesiology, or muscle testing, is a helpful tool for monitoring how your body is responding to changes in lifestyle, such as diet and supplements. If you have never heard of muscle testing, there are natural health providers who can show you how to use it to determine if a product is going to help you, and how much product to take at any given time. It is hard to explain on paper because it is a visual thing. You'll find helpful instructions about how to use kinesiology in the book "Healthy Healing: A Guide to Self-Healing for Everyone," by Linda Rector Page, a naturopathic doctor. Through muscle testing, a body shows and "tells" what it needs. This is a guide to let you know where to start, such as with the liver, gallbladder, kidneys, or other.

A word of caution about health food stores: Many people working in health food stores only know what sales reps have told them about the products they are selling. It is important that you develop reliable relationships with store personnel by asking plenty of questions. First, read labels thoroughly. Then, ask the sales clerk or store owner:

~ Who has purchased this product regularly? What was their experience with it?

~ Is there anyone I might call or write who has experience or information to share about this product?

~ Can you recommend a natural health care provider who can give me direction or information?

Most medical doctors do not get intensive training regarding nutrition. They are not taught what the human body can do to heal itself, or what improvements can be made by simply taking a multivitamin or multimineral.

~ Is there a website for this product?

~ Is there an 800-number listed on the label? If so, call and ask for additional information.

As you work to change your health, a little common sense goes a long way. Pay attention to your body and trust your intuition. Breathe, meditate, or pray. Be patient with yourself! Each unhealthy pattern is like a layer that needs to be peeled back and revealed. Some layers will be more difficult than others and might have an emotional connection that needs attention. Healing your body will also help you heal your life. Be gentle, yet persistent. Remain optimistic. Keep an open heart and mind and you *will* change your health. I promise!

> **You cannot discover new oceans unless you have the courage to lose sight of the shore.**
>
> **Anonymous**

5
NUTRITION & FOOD
Nutrition and medicine are equally important

The human body is a magnetic, electrochemical factory that produces energy. That energy is used to make your heart beat, your eyes blink, and your hair grow. Energy allows you to run from a tiger, solve problems, and bend rules. Your body requires the right fuel in order to perform all its functions. Food is the body's fuel. The right food source is required to help each and every body perform its task. If the fuel you are putting into your body is insufficient, you will get an insufficient reaction. In other words, if you take a gasoline engine and put diesel in it, how well will it run?

The stomach breaks down food into the natural components the body requires. The intestines extract these components for the body's use. The lungs bring in air for an oxygen-carbon exchange with the blood, and the blood distributes the oxygen as well as the nutritional components to all organs and cells via the circulatory system. What your body does not need, the bladder, bowels, skin, lungs, and lymph system eliminate.

The information that follows has been handed down since Hippocrates. Other world cultures have ancient traditions that successfully address basic health needs, illnesses, and diseases. These cultures regard food as medicine. It is important to keep an open mind, a persistent heart, and a searching soul in your quest for better health.

Let's discuss fresh, RAW fruits and vegetables, which contain active enzymes necessary for the assimilation of ALL foods. Without *some* fresh, raw foods in EVERY MEAL, the body will not efficiently extract nutrients from cooked foods.

By the way, cooking foods at high temperatures will eliminate some essential nutrients and enzymes, as does freezing! And, if you use a microwave oven for cooking, you may as well eat the containers and packaging because the microwave process effectively destroys a large part of the nutrients and enzyme values of food. If you give microwaved water to your plants they will die! (I maintain that the radiation process utilized in microwaving is good only for drying newspapers.)

The body requires approximately 97-125 nutrients a day to maintain whole, healthy cells. These nutrients are comprised of approximately 60-75 minerals, 22-25 vitamins, 12 essential amino acids, and 3 essential fatty acids. Without this recipe, a body cannot maintain peak performance while also regenerating 140 billion whole, healthy new cells each and every day.

Why Raw and Organic Foods?

It is essential that the body have the ability to recognize what you are ingesting. Many of the foods in the typical American diet come from a box, a can, a package, or are prepared at high temperatures. Such foods not only are deficient in nutritional value, they also contain chemical additives, preservatives, and colorants that enter the body as particles that the body does not recognize. This requires the immune system to "stop them at the gate" and say, "Wait a moment! You're supposed to be green beans (or apple, or corn on the cob), but there is something not right. You contain foreign chemical components I do not know how to process."

So, the immune system ends up playing gatekeeper, allowing each foreign particle to go its separate way, hoping the body will eliminate them. Think of it this way: the minute you take a bite of food, chew it and swallow it, the food is reduced to its unique chemistry. The apple you eat isn't recognized by the body as an apple. It must be transformed into a digestible, chemical product that the body can recognize and assimilate. If not, it is the same as putting sugar into a gas tank: it gums up the engine so the car won't run properly.

When something unrecognizable enters the body, especially in excess, it overloads the circuits. The circuits (meaning the cells), cannot do their jobs efficiently. Nothing is accomplished and in actuality, normal body functioning becomes more difficult.

The human body is comprised of cells, fluid, magnetics, and electricity. In short, it is all chemistry and it is essential that this chemistry operate in harmony. We need to eliminate foods that upset this chemistry because they contain chemicals and preservatives, or have been altered through processing, freezing, microwaving, or cooking at a high temperature.

Half the foods in most produce departments have been hybridized through genetic alterations. And then there are "GM" foods, those genetically modified to contain traits selected from other species. Do you know which ones? I don't, because details change constantly. By some reports half the potatoes and tomatoes and most of the corn and soy have been genetically altered. Remember too that anything in the produce section that comes in a box, can, or package, contains added preservatives.

Ignore what the label says. Buy a package of "organic" spinach in a plastic bag, pop open the bag and take a big whiff. See if the only thing you smell is spinach. It may be organically grown spinach, but it also may have been sprayed with a chemical gas as a preservative for the bagging process. Once a preservative has been added to enhance shelf life, produce can no longer be considered organic.

Remember: IF YOUR FOOD HAS NO FLAVOR, IT HAS NO NUTRITION. Just one example: the taste of store-bought tomatoes versus tomatoes fresh from the garden.

A word of caution about preservatives. There is evidence that one of the chemicals in sodas, when stored at 87-degrees, turns to formaldehyde, a chemical used for embalming. Personally, I would rather not have my cells loaded with embalming fluid before I am through using them! Don't take my word for it — check it out yourself.

In a perfect world we could all grow our own plants and raise our own animals. In today's world we cannot do that, but there are herbal magazines, organic magazines, and health & healing magazines with information about where to get real organic foods. Check their resource sections for lists of vendors who will ship their organic products to you. If you have friends and neighbors who are interested in buying organic, you can start your own support system for pooling resources and boosting your buying power.

Or, grow your own produce for trade with other like-minded people. Working together, asking questions, and sharing knowledge creates harmony and builds community, all of which contribute to a better and healthier world.

> **You can grow herbs and vegetables in window boxes or patio pots. At the very least, sprout some organic seeds and eat the sprouts. There. You are on your way to healthier eating!**

Free Radicals

A word about free radicals: by definition, a free radical is an atom or a group of atoms with at least one unpaired electron. Free radicals are normally present in small amounts within the body. They are active compounds produced when molecules react with oxygen. The presence of too many free radicals can play a major part in the deterioration within the body.

Damage occurs when excessive free radicals alter the way cells code genetic material. This means the body can be manipulated into thinking that a necessary protein is a foreign substance for the body to destroy. Problems occur when too many of these mutated cells remain in your blood, which itself delivers your body's food supply.

Science has determined that people die prematurely due to free radical damage. I recall what these roaming free radicals look like through a computerized microscope – they resemble a small raindrop with tiny spike-like tentacles. These float through your bloodstream, randomly attacking and mutating healthy cells they encounter. Normally, free radicals only attack diseased or damaged cells, but when there are too many of them they bump into healthy cells and damage them.

The good news is that the body produces natural enzymes to help neutralize free radicals. They're called "antioxidants." We can also counter free radical activity through diet, vitamins, and/or antioxidant supplements. Free radicals thrive on saturated fat molecules and non-organic sugars, the kind found in junk food, fast food, and processed foods.

It makes sense then, for us to reduce our "bad" fat and overindulgent intake of sugars. To resist free radical invasion we should eat unsaturated fats ("good" fats) such as those found in olive oil, avocados, nuts, and seeds. And, natural butter is always a better choice than margarine. Margarine was originally manufactured to fatten commercially raised turkeys. When it began to kill the birds it was reformulated for human consumption. Natural butter can be mixed with extra virgin olive oil or yogurt and a pinch of salt to make a tasty spread.

> **There are dreamers and there are planners. The planners make their dreams come true.**
> **Anonymous**

Antioxidants

Antioxidants are important as they assist in disabling free radical activity. Antioxidants can be found in vitamins A, C, and zinc. They are also contained in liquid berry juices like Alive™, Noni™, Xango™, and Ninja Red™, all of which are rich in antioxidants.

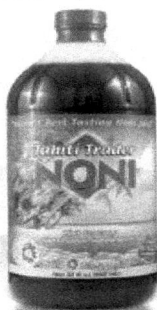

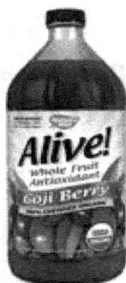

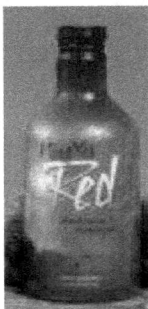

Noni is a fruit used by Polynesian cultures for over 1500 years. It is helpful for degenerative diseases and provides anti-tumor and anti-inflammatory effects. The same applies to Goji and mangosteen (the key to Ninja Red™).

Just be aware that these products can be expensive, and keep in mind that too much of a good thing can become a bad thing. The same is true of antioxidants. Too many can move your health in the wrong direction. Read labels. Consult with a professional. Pay attention to your body and learn to listen to what it is telling you. Common sense, common sense, common sense!

Whole Grains

If grains, especially wheat, bother your digestion, seek help in evaluating whether you might have celiac disease, a serious health challenge.

There is a lot in the press now about whole grains. Many items are called "whole grain" that in truth, are not. Some rules of thumb when purchasing whole grain products:

~ Read the label. Products called "multi-grain" are not necessarily "whole" grain. Whole grains are those that have not been overly milled, and have the original grain, or *kernel*, largely intact.

~ The product should have a minimum of 3 grams of dietary fiber per serving. If it takes more than one serving to get 3 grams of fiber, the product is not whole grain.

~ Any grain that has been baked at 350-degrees no longer has its original vitamins, minerals, amino acids, fatty acids, or enzymes. Benefits are lost at 112-degrees.

One last word about food: If it has no color and no flavor, it has no nutritional value! When you eat foods with no nutritional value, your brain is going to signal, "Feed me, feed me!" Your body, the chemical factory that it is, will still seek nutrition. "Where's the calcium? Where's the vitamin C? Where's the zinc?" In order to satisfy a deficiency of nutrients, the brain will signal you to keep eating. You may not actually be hungry, but undernourished.

Dairy Products

Contrary to popular belief and despite the dairy industry's advertising, a body past weaning does not need milk. Dairy products are not and should not be considered a good source for protein and calcium. Our bodies simply cannot absorb the protein and calcium molecules altered by pasteurization and homogenization.

Humans are the only mammals to consume milk after weaning. According to Dr. Kurt Esselbacher, chairman of the Department of Medicine at the Harvard School of Medicine, tiny undigested fat fragments from homogenized milk pose serious health problems. They are one of the major contributors to heart disease in the United States.

Milk also has a negative effect on both the digestive and immune systems, as it is mucus-forming and acidic. Common symptoms attributed to milk drinkers are cataracts, eczema, allergies, colds, influenza, ear infections, gastric distress, and raised cholesterol levels. Cow's milk was made for calves, not for humans. It has over 20 times more casein (mucus and acid-forming properties) than can be properly utilized by the human body. One study involved feeding pasteurized, homogenized cow's milk to calves. The calves did not survive past 6 weeks.

If you feel you cannot go without the taste of dairy products, consider trying an occasional serving of yogurt, or rice or coconut milk, almond or soy milk, or a mix of them (1/3 each of rice, almond, soy). My best recommendation is little or no milk. Save the little you can have for inclusion in goodies like gravy and sauces. A little is fine; a lot is not.

Acid vs. Alkaline

Science tells us that disease cannot thrive in your body if you have a slightly alkaline pH. The blood is always slightly alkaline, the saliva and urine are slightly acidic. Picture the pH of your saliva and urine as battery acid dropped onto your trousers. A little acid eats a small hole in your pants. A lot of acid will eat not only through your pants, but your skin as well. This is what goes on inside your body.

We know that an overly acidic pH causes cellular breakdown and creates the perfect environment for disease to take hold of your body. pH testing kits for urine and saliva can be purchased at pharmacies and health food stores. 6.5 to 6.9 is a natural pH for both urine and saliva. To test your saliva, spit into a paper cup and dip the test strip into it. The paper will turn a color. Compare that color to the indicators on the package to get a number. That number should be as close to 7.0 as possible. To test urine, follow a similar procedure. (See Resources in the back of this book for my favorite pH testing kit.)

As you work on changing your diet, it will help if you keep a log or journal listing each of these pH test numbers and the time of day you administered the test. If you test your first urine and saliva every morning, you'll get an idea of what is going on in your body all night long. During an acidic night, not much repair work takes place, and in fact, there is more destruction of cells occurring than construction. Remember, cells are always destructing and constructing. Healthy cell construction keeps aging at bay.

Practitioners of natural healing teach that if you have slightly alkaline or natural 7.0 pH, you are less likely to be susceptible to disease. No matter what the disease – cancer, arthritis, or insomnia – chances are its symptoms stem from an acidic pH condition. That means every cell in your body is struggling to stay alive, trying to function while being eaten up (similar to the battery acid on your trousers). Cells cannot be effective under these conditions.

In the standard American diet, acidic foods tend to comprise the majority of food on the plate. Meat, potatoes, bread, pasta, desserts, soda, and alcohol are all acidic. It is the vegetable kingdom that is alkaline. Between 75-99% of all veggies are alkaline. For that reason, I recommend that your meals be comprised of 80% alkaline foods. That leaves only 20% for acidic foods. You may want to test your pH before meals to determine what to eat for each meal. If you are in a highly acidic state, you will want to avoid introducing additional acid into your system.

Which foods are alkalizing? Again, 75-99% of vegetables are alkalinizing foods and 50-75% of all fruits are alkaline.

Acidifiers include lack of sleep, overwork, worry, tension, anger, jealousy, resentment.

Acid remedy – drink one teaspoon molasses mixed with one tablespoon raw apple cider vinegar in 6 oz. of hot water. You can add honey or raw, natural maple syrup to taste. Drink 1 to 10 doses a day.

> **Drinking 1 ounce of aloe vera (liquid or gel) per day for three months will lower LDL (harmful) cholesterol and triglycerides by 40-80%. That could mean it reverses atherosclerosis and heart disease!**
>
> **Be sure the product you buy contains a high level of pure aloe vera, preferably gel.**
>
> **A label reading "100% aloe" is not an assurance of purity.**

Sometimes the acid or alkaline properties of a food change under certain conditions. It is almost always better to consume food products that are as close to how God made them as possible. Vinegars are a good example. They have traditionally been considered acidic, however, raw apple cider vinegar, the one with sediment in the bottom of the bottle, has an alkalizing response in your body that will help the body to heal. So there are certain conditions that can move a food from the acid list to the alkaline list, and vice-versa.

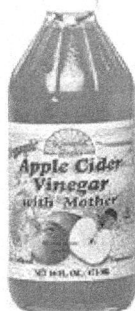

Raw Organic Apple cider vinegar (any brand) is a health tonic with over 30 important nutrients. It contains natural antibiotic and antifungal properties. To use as a detoxifying agent mix 1 tablespoon apple cider vinegar with 1 teaspoon maple syrup and warm water. Drink 1 to 10 doses daily. The key is *unfiltered* apple cider vinegar, which has visible sediment at the bottom. Shown above is just one brand; there are many others.

Eggs are a good example of foods that can be either acidic or alkaline. Eggs technically are an animal protein, and all animal proteins are acidic. Regular store-bought eggs are very acidic at 4.5-5.1 pH. However, organic free-range eggs have a pH of 6.8-6.9, which is still acidic but only slightly. If you cook free-range eggs into an omelet with vegetables, the alkaline properties of the vegetables will offset the acid and reduce its impact on the body.

Yogurt is another good example. Plain yogurt is full of friendly bacteria and is alkalizing. However, most of the yogurt on grocery shelves is the "fruit at the bottom" variety, or is colored, flavored, or sweetened to such an extent that it becomes acidic. To get maximum goodness from the friendly bacteria in the yogurt, and the alkalizing effect you are after, it is better to start with plain yogurt, adding berries and B-grand maple syrup.

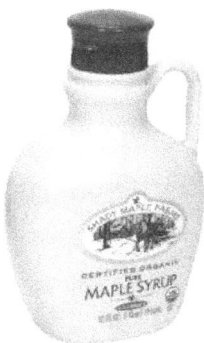

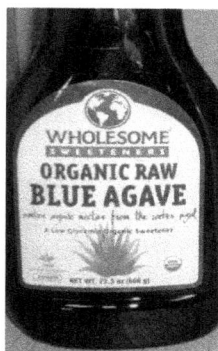

Speaking of B-grade maple syrup, the only other alkalizing sweeteners are Stevia and honey (preferably honey grown in the area where you live). B-grade maple syrup has stronger maple flavor but is richer in nutrients than A-grade.

Instead of white sugars or sugar substitutes, try agave nectar or B-grade maple syrup. B-grade has more nutrition than A-grade. All grades of syrup are treated by the body as a nutritional package, not a "sugar load." Your brain uses more glycogens (sugars) than any other body part. Nutrient-rich glycogens power the brain better.

Keep in mind, too, that the spices you use have alkaline or acidic properties. Fresh herbs that are alkalizing include parsley, sage, rosemary, thyme, cilantro, garlic, and onions. As for salt, it is preferable to use sea salt because the fluids in your body are a lot more like ocean water than anything else.

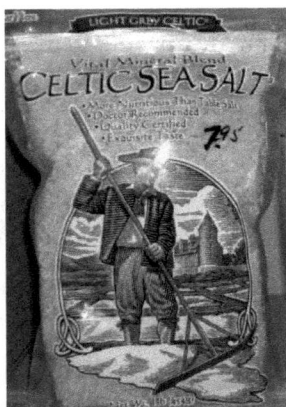

Sea salts have a much better response within the body chemistry than table salts. Every cell has a sodium-potassium pump. If our sodium levels decline or are way below normal range, cells stop pumping. Shown is just one brand of many sea salts available.

Curry and turmeric are alkaline seasonings. Turmeric is also considered anti-inflammatory.

Inflammation from an injury, like an ankle sprain with swelling, serves a purpose. It is like God's bubble wrap, protecting the tissue through partial immobilization to avoid further injury. However, when there is inflammation due to infection, or the body is hyperacidic, the swollen tissues are trying to protect themselves from the acid. They swell up, taking room from other cells. Some people take turmeric as a supplement to offset a state of inflammation.

Aspirin

A word about aspirin and the popular saying, "An aspirin a day keeps the doctor away." The negative effects of aspirin can outweigh the positive. Aspirin and aspirin-type anti-inflammatory painkillers, when used routinely, destroy vital nutrients (like vitamin C) which the body uses to repair cells.

Aspirin also lowers potassium levels, which offsets the mineral balance, accelerating the destruction of cartilage and setting into motion the breakdown of the gastrointestinal lining. The result: ulcers. Aspirin, when taken during pregnancy, can affect the fetus's blood, and has been linked to stillbirth.

Regular aspirin was originally made from white willow bark. White willow is a tree whose bark contains beneficial compounds. But when altered in the laboratory to remove some of its elements, the resultant standard aspirin pill will irritate your stomach. This is the difference between natural organic products and manmade products. However, do not expect a pharmaceutical response from white willow bark like you would get from aspirin. The herb may work slower or require a higher dosage. Try taking the recommended dosage on the bottle, then pay attention to your symptoms to determine what works for you. If you experiment a little, or muscle test yourself, you will be better able to determine the amount you need to take.

A sign that aspirin-type products are not for you could be such symptoms as ringing in your ears or an upset stomach. This is one way the body communicates its need for less medication and stress, or more nutrients and less stress.

There are other "painkillers" from the herb kingdom. They don't actually kill the pain, but rather feed your nervous system so that it can better handle stress. These herbs include:

~ Chamomile, hops, marjoram
~ Skullcap, kava kava
~ Lavender, lily, gardenia scents
~ Young Living™ brand oils

Use singly or combine them until you discover a formula that works. Plus, there are other herbs for pain relief. Reading and research will lead you to them.

Antacids

One definition of an antacid is an agent that neutralizes acidity, especially acidity in the digestive tract. If you need antacids regularly, the foods you are eating are all wrong for your digestive juices.

Antacids are the most common over-the-counter medication sold in the United States. Examples include aluminum hydroxide and magnesium oxide. Calcium carbonate antacids such as Tums™, Alka-2™, etc., actually produce a rebound effect on gastric acid secretion and may contribute to the formation of kidney stones.

Antacids generally reduce hydrochloric acid (HCL) in the stomach and prevent the digestion of protein. They neutralize acids that cause fermentation, but they also reduce natural HCL production. This is harmful because more HCL is needed to treat the cause of disease rather than the symptoms.

Excessive use of antacids results in a deficiency of certain minerals, which in turn results in low HCL levels. Low HCL levels cause over-alkalinity in the blood – or alkalosis.

The sodium bicarbonate antacids such as Rolaids™, Alka-Seltzer™, Bromo-Seltzer™, etc., have a tendency to induce systemic alkalosis and to interfere with heart and kidney function.

The aluminum/magnesium compounds such as Maalox™, Mylanta™, Di-gel™, etc., cause calcium and phosphorous depletion, as well as causing aluminum toxicity and/or accumulation of aluminum in the brain.

Alkalosis is caused when foods are not properly digested. Instead of reaching for the over-the-counter drugs like Pepcid AC™, Alka-Seltzer™, or the pink stuff, try ... ginger!

Ginger
~ Is cheaper, has no side effects, and is actually *good* for your stomach and digestive tract.
~ Increases the production of natural substances that protect the stomach lining and provides an anti-ulcer effect.
~ Has been used for centuries and is best known for its effect on nausea. This includes morning sick-

ness, motion sickness, and nausea resulting from anesthesia.

~ Enhances the muscular activity of the stomach and intestines.

~ Stimulates the gall bladder, which enhances digestion.

~ Is used throughout the world for treating and preventing gastrointestinal diseases.

~ Is an anti-inflammatory, and is used for musculoskeletal ailments, like arthritis, bursitis, sore muscles, etc.

~ Is used as a cardio tonic (heart tonic). Ginger's effect on the body is considered key to preventing both angina pain and risk of heart attack by maintaining a strong, steady pulse.

Peppermint tea(s) are also a great remedy for digestive upset – not peppermint flavoring (or extract), but tea. Or try a few drops of peppermint essential oil in water.

> **The quality of a person's life is in direct proportion to his or her commitment to excellence.**
> **Anonymous**

Tonic Herbs

Herbs that help in situations where antacids would be used are called "tonic herbs." Tonic herbs are just that – a tonic for the whole body, working primarily with the digestive system. These herbs sharpen the appetite, promote better waste elimination, aid in digestion, soothe the stomach, and gradually build strength, energy and overall health. They invigorate, refresh, and strengthen every organ in the body. This list of tonic herbs provides a starting point:

~ Barberry

~ Golden Seal (Can be harsh on the liver; check with a professional)

~ Peruvian Bark

~ White Poplar

~ European Centaury

~ Blessed Thistle

~ Myrrh, or Gum Myrrh

~ Balmony

~ Gentian

~ Red Clover

~ Pau d' Arco

~ Swedish Bitters

Swedish bitters derive from a 500-year-old European remedy to rejuvenate vital organs, improve regularity, aid digestion, and cleanse internal systems. Use 2 to 6 drops in warm water or tea, drunk 2 to 6 times daily, especially just before or after meals.

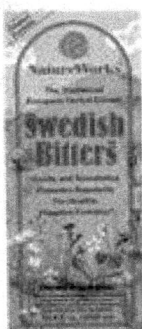

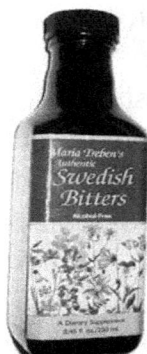

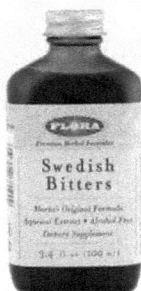

The recipe for Swedish bitters is credited to Dr. Phillipus Paracelus, a Swiss physician who lived in the mid-16th century. Its combination of herbs aids digestion, improving absorption of nutrients so that all cells are better fed and hydrated. It functions as an alternative to typical antacids.

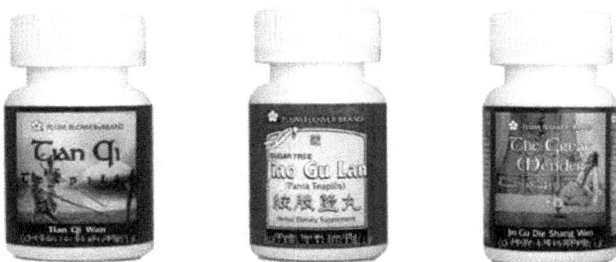

Plum Flower is the company making 6000-year-old formulas. These are three of my favorites: Above left: Tian Qi™ is a blood clot dissolver; Center: Jiao Gu Lan™ is an overall body rejuvenator for anti-aging; Right: The Great Mender™ helps fix, mend, and repair bone, flesh and cartilage.

> **Ask any wise man what he desires**
> **and he will answer: more wisdom.**
> **Anonymous**

6
VITAMINS, MINERALS, SUPPLEMENTS

I have discovered over the years that rather than working piecemeal, if you start with a multivitamin + multimineral supplement you will have greater luck in giving the body everything it requires. Think of it this way: If a contractor needs nails but has to wait for somebody else to supply them, he is delayed in his work. This is also true of the healing process. If the body already has the "nails" it needs for reconstruction, it can work more efficiently. Vitamins and minerals will not cure anything. They provide your body the proper tools (nutrient chemistry) to heal itself the way it is programmed to do.

A multivitamin/multimineral can give you the necessary components on hand so that when the body needs them, there they are. I recommend liquid multis because they are more easily digested and assimilated than capsules or tablets. Besides, some of the tablets out there are so loaded with binders and fillers that they cannot dissolve before elimination occurs. This is a particular problem for the elderly, whose systems are in a weakened condition and/or are out of balance. The pill actually comes out the other end. Sometimes it is so un-dissolved that you can clearly read what it was!

Following are just some of the liquid vitamin-mineral products I've found. Liquids always absorb more completely than nutrients in pill form, especially if you slosh them around in your mouth before swallowing.

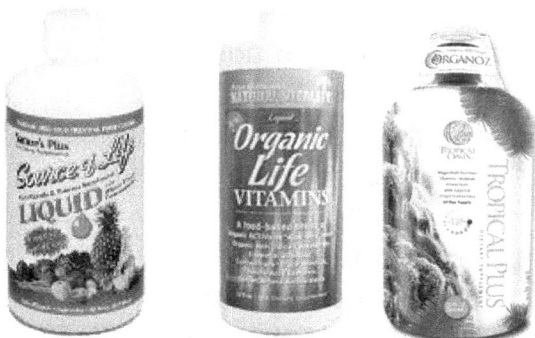

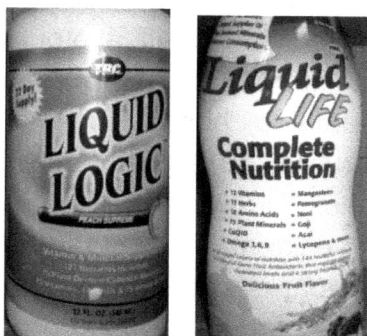

Absorption in the mouth bypasses a compromised intestinal tract, and saliva contains enzymes essential for the assimilation of nutrients. The mucosal lining and the big blue veins under your tongue absorb nutrients immediately; no waiting for absorption to occur in the digestive system.

Naturopaths and health & healing advocates recommend you actually chew your liquids for maximum absorption. However, if you have an aversion to strong tastes you may need to take supplements in pill form. Focus your awareness on whether such pills are being broken down for assimilation by your system. I have some clients taking 45-55 pills and tablets a day, and some of them notice un-dissolved tablets exiting the "other end." This indicates a lack of digestion. Because the tablets did not break down, the body did not get the maximum benefit.

Most nutrients will not interfere with your prescription medications unless your Rx dictates "not to be taken with foods." These nutrients *are* foods. They will work better if you take them at different times than your prescribed or OTC medications. For more information, you can ask the staff at your vitamin store whether they can identify any known contraindications for the supplement you choose.

We must be willing to experiment. Human bodies are like snowflakes. No two are alike. You will need to be patient and diligent. The cleaner your internal body, the better your overall health. The more natural and organic the nutrients you absorb and assimilate, the faster your body will heal and the sooner you will feel great.

Rotation is the name of the game. When you have used a product for 3 months or so, switch to another quality brand so that your body perceives the new benefits to be had therein.

Vitamins

Vitamins are like spark plugs for the body. You cannot live on vitamins; they are not substitutes for food. Instead, they stimulate nutrition. As catalysts, they work on the cellular level, often as co-enzymes, regulating metabolic processes through enzyme activity to convert protein and carbohydrates into tissue and energy.

Vitamins are absolutely necessary for growth, vitality, and resistance to disease through healthy aging. It is impossible to sustain life without them. Even when a body is "running out" of a certain vitamin, the resulting problems may be hard to pinpoint because the cells usually continue to function with decreasing efficiency. Eventually they will either suffer severe damage or else receive proper nutrition.

Vitamin supplements will fill these nutritional gaps at the deepest levels. Regenerative changes in body chemistry usually require as much time to rebuild as they did to decline. Supplemental vitamins not only help us heal, but can also help us advance beyond average health to optimal health.

According to naturopathic doctor Linda Rector, Ph.D., "Even as basic as the RDA [recommended daily allowances] are, not one dietary survey has shown that Americans consume anywhere near the suggested RDA amounts in their normal diets."

In one USDA survey, not one of the 21,500 participants consumed 100% of the RDA nutrient recommendations over a 3-day period. Only 3% ate the recommended number of servings of each of the four food groups, and only 12% ate the RDA of protein, calcium, iron, magnesium, zinc, and vitamins. It is pretty safe to say that *everyone* can benefit from taking a multivitamin/multimineral supplement.

Minerals

Every cell in the body uses minerals for every function. Minerals are responsible for the osmosis of cellular liquids, electrical activity in the nervous system, and most metabolic functions. Minerals transport oxygen through the systems of the body, govern heartbeats, help us sleep, and are major factors dealing with mental and emotional balance.

Minerals are also essential to every single movement, twitch, itch, cell division, reproduction, bone formation, digestion of food, and for maintaining a slightly alkaline pH (which is just as it should be).

There are seven major minerals: calcium, chlorine, magnesium, phosphorus, potassium, sodium, and sulphur. All other are "trace" minerals. TRC-brand Liquid Logic Vitamin & Minerals ™ supplement states that "plant derived minerals should not be confused with metallic minerals which come from clay, ground up rocks and soil, sea water, or come from the Great Salt Lake."

Trace minerals are only .01% of body weight, yet deficiencies in these micronutrients can cause severe depression, PMS and menstrual disorders, hyperactivity in children, sugar imbalances (hypoglycemia and diabetes), unnatural stress responses, high blood pressure, osteoporosis, premature aging, memory loss, and the inability to heal quickly.

Minerals cannot be synthesized by the body and must come from the food we eat, mineral hot springs and baths (absorption through the skin), or from herbs and supplements.

I use liquid multivitamin/multimineral supplements since they are what the body absorbs best. Make certain you get what your body needs. Choose a product with a minimum of 60 minerals.

> **Every cell in your body uses minerals for every function.**
> **Give your body what it needs to operate smoothly and heal itself.**

Herbs & Supplements

Today's American diet of refined foods, an abundance of animal proteins, too much caffeine, and unnatural food fats, inhibits mineral absorption. When life's ups and downs put us in a position to rely on tobacco, alcohol, steroids, antibiotics, and drugs (including OTC varieties), we can experience a depleted mineral state.

Compounding this is the fact that many minerals and trace minerals are no longer sufficiently present in our fruits and vegetables, and the foods that are mineral-rich are costly and either low in quality or quantity.

Organically grown, unsprayed produce is hard to find, difficult to keep fresh, and expensive to purchase. Luckily, we can turn to herbs and supplements to provide us the nutrients we need. It's no secret that herbs can help improve the quality of our health. In fact, there are more than 100 different species of herbs available, and many of today's wonder drugs are derived from them. It would be hard to overestimate the healing power of fresh organic herbs such as parsley, cilantro, sage, basil, thyme, and rosemary. When using fresh herbs in cooked dishes, add them as a "finish" in the last few minutes, as heat destroys some of their nutritional properties. You can find out more about herbs as natural medicine by reading reference books such as those mentioned in early chapters or in my list on page 92.

Remember: Whether you choose liquid supplements, capsules, tablets, or powders, it is important that all supplements be organic and of high quality. Organic liquid vitamins and minerals can be purchased at any health food or vitamin store. Formulations may include capsules that contain low-temperature dried organic herbs, fruits, or vegetables, with live enzymes.

What did I say about rotation? For the best long-term results, rotate to another quality brand of supplement every 2-3 months.

The human body is an organic environment, or what I call "God-made." When you give the body "manmade" products you are introducing chemistry that the body cannot use and might not rid itself of. If the supplement is fabricated and synthetic, it is unlikely your body will have the capacity to utilize much of it. It is a certainty that your system will not utilize a synthetic substance with the same efficiency as one originating from an organic source. This is because organics have comparable chemistry to the body, providing a harmonizing, balancing effect. In opposition, synthetics are like "dirty chemistry." They result in the body having to defend itself against foreign, confusing, and often unrecognizable substances.

When beginning a new vitamin/mineral regimen, keep in mind that it takes 90 days for your conscious mind to catch up to your cellular changes. In other words, you may not notice changes for 90 days! Every system in the body is INTERDEPENDENT upon every other system. If the body is lacking a nutrient, it will be harder for all other nutrients to work. Since every cell in your body connects to every other cell, the body's components cannot work without communicating. All of the body's chemistry must work in close harmony for the body to build and maintain optimum performance.

There are elements in the herbal kingdom that automatically contain a "grouping" of nutrients. This is why green beans grown in a poor soil will not have the nutrition or the depth of taste of green beans grown in herbicide-free, nutrient-rich soil. This is the case with herbs, too.

Thus the development of what is called "standardization." Manufacturers have taken nutrient-poor herbs and blended them with nutrient-rich herbs. In natural medicine, herb gatherers call this "wild crafting." They automatically collect the same variety of herb from all four directions of a hill's sides (north/east/south/west) and blend them together. When you blend different qualities of the same herb together, nutrient-rich harmony results. Native healers teach this ancient Asian healing protocol. When we give the body high quality food and supplements we provide ourselves a higher potential for maximum absorption, increasing the potential for optimum health and healing. Herbs have always been one of the best medicines.

> **A procrastinator is never bothered by the little things that plague the rest of us.**
> **He always waits until they grow into big things!**

Garlic

Garlic has been used to treat everything from abscesses to whooping cough. The list includes colds, fever, flu symptoms, coughs, earache, bronchitis, shortness of breath, sinus congestion, headache, high blood pressure, arteriosclerosis, hypertension, athlete's foot fungus, diarrhea, dysentery, gout, rheumatism, pinworms, old ulcers, and snakebites. Garlic is considered an anti-microbial (kills microbes) and is recommended for people with cancer and heart disease.

According to the Herb Research Foundation in Boulder Colorado, the aromatic part of the garlic is *allicin*, which is strongly antibacterial. However, allicin is lost when garlic is heated. Eating it raw is the only way to keep the allicin active. Raw garlic is effective in combating the herpes virus and Candida (yeast). It works on antibiotic-resistant bacteria as well. Allicin has shown the strongest antimicrobial effect.

Hippocrates recommended garlic as a diuretic, to regulate digestion, to alleviate bowel pain, inflammation, running sores, and to regulate menstruation.

Garlic can be taken as a tea, or capsules can be made by grinding dried garlic cloves. Odorless formulations don't have the same medical power because the smelly part of garlic is the allicin. I have chewed a clove a day for years, chased by warm water. The aroma goes away after I drink liquid chlorophyll. Some alternatives to garlic include tea tree oil, GSE, and olive leaf.

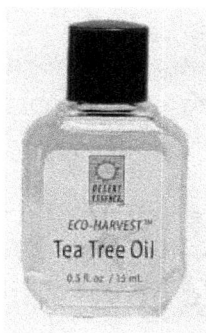

Used topically, this essential oil from Australia is an antiseptic and antifungal. Used by indigenous people for centuries for boils, cuts, scrapes, earache, hair and scalp problems, scabies, warts, insect bites, athlete's foot, and acne. Added to water it becomes a gargle for sore throats and mouth sores.

Advice about tea tree oil is against swallowing it. However, I've had people tell me they mix a few drops with water to take for upset stomach or heartburn.

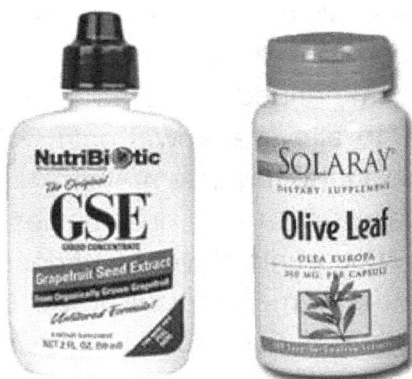

Grapefruit seed extract is a natural antibiotic, working against yeast infection, diarrhea, infected cuts, gingivitis, strep throat, ringworm, and ear and nail infections.

Olive leaf comes in capsules and extract. It is antibacterial, antiviral, antifungal, anti-parasite, and an antioxidant. Treats over 120 illnesses.

> **Use what talents you possess.**
> **The woods would be very silent**
> **if no birds sang except those that**
> **sang best.**

Chlorophyll & "Green Drinks"

Included in your daily diet of nutrients should be one of the "green drinks." There are about 5 or 6 main green drinks: blue-green algae, spirulina, Green-Magma™, and wheat grass juice, etc. Each of these contains the "lifeblood" of plants – chlorophyll.

One product I recommend is liquid chlorophyll, which is also available at the health food store. Known to most herbalists as "Nature's green healer," chlorophyll's chemistry is so close to our own blood that it makes me wonder why science hasn't figured out a way to use it orally as a blood booster. It is the cleanest, purest, freshest blood tonic I can think of!

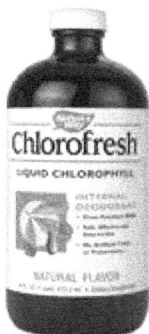

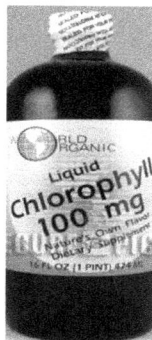

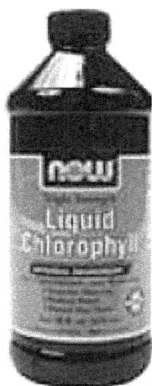

Chlorophyll is very similar to human blood. It detoxifies the liver and is an antioxidant. It calms nerves and alleviates insomnia. Each formula will taste different. As always, rotate through brands — don't stick with just one.

Human blood contains a red pigment with a web of carbon, hydrogen, oxygen, and nitrogen atoms grouped around a single atom of iron. Chlorophyll contains a green pigment with a similar web of the same atoms, except that at its center is a single atom of magnesium.

Research scientist E. Bircher calls chlorophyll, "concentrated sun power," and says, "Chlorophyll increases the function of the heart, has a positive effect on the vascular system, the intestines, the uterus and the lungs."

Liquid chlorophyll has valuable antiseptic qualities and yet is soothing and healing to all tissues. A daily dose of 1 ounce or more is beneficial for the prevention of high blood pressure, arthritis, and arteriosclerosis. The directions on the bottle will say to take 1-2 tablespoons, but I suggest 2-4 ounces daily … and green poop is good!

Greens in general hold more nutritional value than most other foods on the planet. They are loaded with necessary enzymes and nutrients. Liquid chlorophyll is typically the juice of alfalfa. Alfalfa is the most nutritionally rich land plant because its roots can extend up to six feet into the earth, absorbing more nutrients from the soil. Deep soil has not been exposed to pollution in the air, pesticides, etc., and is therefore more nutrient-rich. Remember: If the soil has no nutrients, neither will the food!

Oxi Chlor™ brand liquid chlorophyll, which comes in an eyedropper bottle, derives from nettles, which contains different nutrients than the alfalfa products. It is not as nutrient-rich as the others and is commonly used to treat liver problems. Consider rotating it into your green drink regimen.

There are at least 4-6 different high-quality brands of liquid chlorophyll. Look for one that provides at least 100 mg per dose so that you get the most bang for your buck. Some brands, like World Organics™, add other complimentary elements such as aloe and alatonin.

The other green products – spirulina, blue-green algae, Supragreen Magma™, etc., come in liquid, powder, or pill form, and derive from different sources.

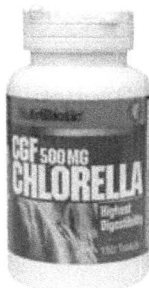

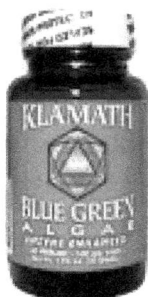

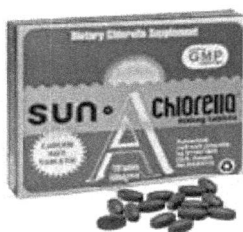

All greens help our bodies heal because they are rich in nutrients, protein, fiber, vitamins, minerals, and enzymes. They help the immune system, accelerate healing and tissue repair, strengthen the liver, reduce the stiffness of arthritis, normalize blood pressure, and provide energy.

Make sure that the products you choose are organic and not fabricated in a laboratory.

Research has discovered that the best results come when liquid multivitamin/multiminerals and green nutrients are taken throughout the day rather than at one sitting. If your body is not well, or if you are experiencing the effects of cellular breakdown, ingesting these products throughout the day will give your system the consistent support necessary to heal.

You can be secure in knowing there is NO chance whatsoever of overdose. These supplements are foods. What your body doesn't use it will eliminate. The combination of all the organic liquid nutrients consumed one after the other in combination with whole, fresh foods, creates a complete and balanced nutritional foundation.

I myself drink 1/3 bottle of chlorophyll per day for prevention and maintenance. I like to alternate between the alfalfa and nettle-derived chlorophylls, and other varieties of green supplements. You can try my approach: put 2 to 4 ounces into a bottle of water and sip it throughout the day until it is gone. I rotate brands and formulas because I believe God gave us a rotation diet in the form of seasonally available foods. As a natural healer I like to follow the rhythms of Mother Nature. The rotation of vitamins and supplements is in harmony with those cycles.

Even though we now can get all foods at any time in the form of canned, frozen, or packaged, this does not mean it is right or natural for us to consume them.

Seasonal foods have properties that are appropriate to the season in which they are abundant and available. Our bodies have seasonally appropriate chemistries that prepare and assist us to utilize these nutrients for the maximum overall benefit.

For example, some of the winter foods are more substantial and contain more fat so that they help us maintain body heat, keeping us warm during frigid weather. On the other hand, summer foods are cooling, lighter, and easier to digest so that they minimize the body's workload in the heat of the day.

Following the rotational diet with your supplements is beneficial in the same way. Let me explain: I have found that for most people, a new diet program works great for the first 2 ½ to 3 months. This might happen to you. What happens is your body hits a plateau where the new food plan seems to no longer work. This is because your body has ingested the elements of the new diet, progressing in cellular to the next "rung" on the "health ladder." Your body is now healthier than before the introduction of the new dietary elements.

Since your biochemical body has changed and become healthier, the only way your body can signal that it is time to move to the next level, is to plateau. So a plateau doesn't indicate that something is breaking down, but rather that you are ready to rotate and introduce new elements to your body. Those of you who are trying to lose or gain weight will experience more success at changing your metabolic rate and weight by changing your nutritional program every 2-½ to 3 months.

My experience is that a rotation diet is beneficial and a practice I recommend to my clients regardless of their particular health challenges. Rotate foods that are seasonably appropriate. Rotate the supplements and vitamins you take. Or, if you are going to continue with a particular formulation of supplement or vitamin, rotate to another brand.

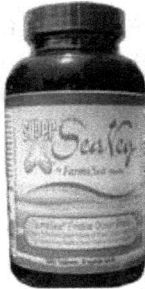

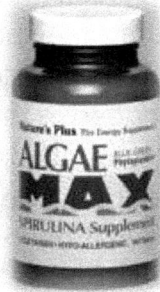

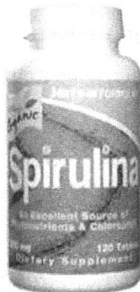

Like other "green foods" and supplements, these also cleanse the liver and feed the body. All greens are good for every cell in our body.

What are Blood Cleansers and who needs them?
Blood cleansers are herbs and foods that help the body remove the "sludge," or toxins and natural waste products, from the blood and lymph systems. They

are important to use because each and every day we are exposed to more toxins and chemical pollution than ever before. We breathe it. We eat it. We drink it. We bathe in it. We walk in it. We work in it.

Since the 1990s, our bodies are no longer clear or clean enough to fight off the onslaught of chemicals we encounter on a daily basis. When our blood and lymph systems are clean, there is nothing for "invaders" to feed on. Less food for the invaders means less reproduction of damaged or diseased cells. Damaged, mutated, or diseased cells are the foundation for both minor and major illnesses ranging from infections to cancer. Blood cleansers have a positive effect on the entire blood system, the heart, veins, arteries, capillaries, and circulation as a whole.

Herbs used primarily to cleanse the blood and lymph systems include:

~ Alfalfa
~ Burdock Root
~ Chaparral
~ Dandelion
~ Echinacea
~ Garlic
~ Onion
~Yellow Dock
~ Red Clover
~ Pau d' Arco
~ Liquid Chlorophyll (Also strengthens weakened organs and tissues)

Dosage:
~ Fresh or dried herb tea –

~ 2 ounces fresh or 1 ounce dried herbs.

~ Stir into 6-8 ounces hot water.

~ Place a lid on the container to keep the volatile oils from escaping.

~ Drink 1-6 cups a day, depending on the severity of symptoms, for 6 days in a row. Take the 7th day off, and then begin again until symptoms are alleviated.

Optional: add licorice root, ginger, or peppermint for taste.

Capsules –

~ As with tea, take for 6 days then rest on the 7th day.

~ Resume again in the same pattern until symptoms are alleviated.

Essiac, Flor Essence, and Hoxsey

Some other products are for people who have serious ongoing conditions like HIV, cancer, chronic fatigue, and Lyme's disease, to name a few. The first is "Essiac™." I also recommend the book, "Essiac Story," which discusses Flor Essence and Essiac. Essiac is a recipe handed down from the Ojibwa Indians of Canada to Rene Caisse, a nurse. Caisse developed the product recipe and administered it to many people with cancer from the 1920s through the 1940s, with significant success. The formula contains burdock root, slippery elm, sheep sorrel, Indian rhubarb, and turkey rhubarb. These herbs work effectively to:

~ Assist the body in cleaning out waste materials.

~ Assist in cleaning out materials no longer needed.

~ Assist the body to feed itself and absorb nutrients.
~ Assist in healing.
I call Essiac a "cleaning-and-feeding-that-helps-you-heal" recipe!

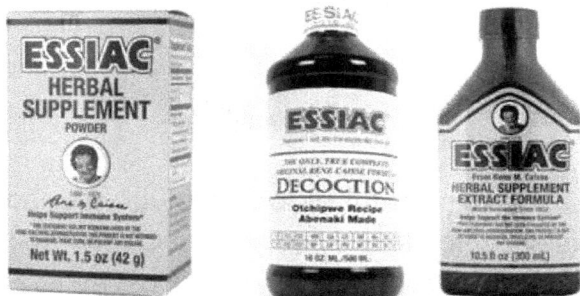

Flor Essence is the next progression from Essiac as it is a stronger formula containing 8 herbs. It contains the same 4 as Essiac plus 4 more cleansing and feeding herbs. Both Essiac and Flor Essence come in the form of capsules, dried powders, tablets, and liquids. By now you know I prefer the liquid form. Some people make a tea, but be aware that tea is the *weakest* form to ingest these products so you may need to increase the package's recommended dosage to receive the desired results.

Be aware that some companies manufacturing Essiac spell it differently. For example, one Canadian company calls their product "CAN essiac." Also, one company makes a capsulated formula and cannot call it Essiac tea (since it's in powdered form), so they label it "ET." Flor Essence is only available from a company named Flora.

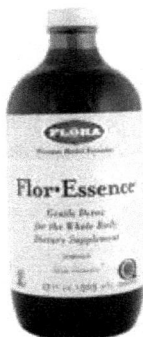

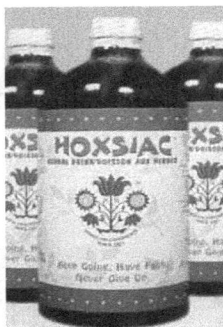

There is another useful herbal formula, named for Harry Hoxsey, who developed a formula for cancer patients in the 1920s through 1930s. Hoxsey is a 12-15 herb formula, so it is stronger yet than the 4-herb Essiac and the 8-herb Flor Essence.

I recommend all three formulations, but not concurrently. The regimen I recommend is as follows, but play with the dosages. If they are too strong, cut back:

~ Start with Essiac (4-herb formula) for 2 ½ to 3 months. It is the mildest formula which works gently.

~ Next switch to Flor Essence (8-herb formula) for 2 ½ to 3 months.

~ Move then to Hoxsey (12-herb formula) for 2 ½ to 3 months.

~ Start the cycle over, but at higher dosages for each formula (because you have moved up the healing ladder). REMEMBER: 6 DAYS ON, THEN THE 7th DAY OFF, so as not to overwhelm your body.

You can use these products in addition to your vitamin/mineral and herbal formulas, and the chlorophyll, though I do not recommend blending them in the same jar as each already has a unique flavor you may not enjoy. Generally speaking, I like some kind of chaser to deal with the taste. Pomegranate juice, which is high in antioxidants, is my favorite. There are also herbal teas like red clover (for one example) that help mediate the taste of herb formulas.

Please note: If your body is severely out of balance, when you start to cleanse, your waste material may not leave the body as quickly as it should and you may feel worse before feeling better, which, in my opinion, is a positive sign that your system is beginning to cleanse itself.

Pay close attention to what your bodily reactions are, though sometimes "negative" reactions are the desired result! For example, if a supplement gives you diarrhea, your body may be ridding itself of dead cells, bi-products, or debris. It is like adding more material to an already full trash can; the garbage will spill over the top!

If you are taking a new supplement or remedy and perceive a "negative" response, sit down and ask yourself whether this is part of the elimination process and the body cleansing itself. Or, did you take too much, causing it to work too hard, too fast in your system? Do you need to adjust the dosage by taking less of the supplement? Is the regimen working for your lifestyle, today? How are you feeling, and if it is for your eventual healing, can you afford to go through the day not feeling particularly well?

Common sense goes a long way with "God's medicines!" The trick is that when you give a body what it needs for health and healing, part of the healing process is to kick out diseased and damaged cells in any way it can. If it is easier for the body to rid itself of those cells through the throat or out through your mouth, as in vomiting or coughing up mucus, then it will do that. If, on the other hand, the undesirable waste is closer to the anus and creates diarrhea, then that is the direction the elimination will take.

Some people will start sweating, which is also a good response because your skin is one of the biggest elimination systems, covering the entire body. Sweating isn't automatically a "bad" reaction. Again, keep in mind that you may not notice the positive changes for 90 days.

Elimination

While we are on the subject, let's talk about elimination. Only 10% of our elimination occurs through the bowel. This is why it is a big deal when people have only one bowel movement per day, especially when you couple that with a habit of shallow breathing, plus preservatives, additives, and coloring in food, plus fluorescent lighting, plus Teflon or formaldehyde in your carpet and chlorine in your water. The equation adds up to an abundance of waste material that is entering the body, and very little that is consistently being eliminated. This causes congestion. This causes blockages. This causes cells to swim in their own waste.

If you are not having a bowel movement from 20 minutes to 1 hour after each meal, then you have a systemic, body-wide garbage strike taking place in your body.

It has been reported that most Americans continuously have between 5 to 20 pounds of fecal matter trapped in their tubal accordion (bowel) at any given time. So, if your bowel movements are not regular, you are experiencing some degree of build-up, or impaction, in your bowel.

The bowel is a long, tubal accordion with a lot of nooks and crannies that can trap acidic and impacted fecal matter. Irritable bowel syndrome, leaky gut syndrome, Crohn's disease, and diverticulitis are all conditions that involve a low-functioning bowel; waste is not eliminating.

In this case, prevention is worth a pound of cure. Animals will actually eat certain foods to unblock their bowel. "National Geographic" magazine reports that birds will clean themselves out by using a reed to give themselves an enema. I'd rather use aloe vera gel! It is one of the best bowel remedies because not only does it help everything slide and glide out of your body, but it also coats the tissues so that the acidity of bowel material won't keep irritating, or eating holes in, the lining of the bowel. Aloe vera gel provides the best value because you can adjust its dilution to fit your needs.

Breathing

Now let's talk about oxygen. Breathe deeply in and out. Every cell in your body requires food, water, and oxygen. Seventy percent of your body's waste is eliminated through your lungs, and it's free!

How you breathe is important. There are two kinds of breathing. Shallow breathing only partially fills the lungs. Shallow breathers have a tendency to be tense, maybe a bit high strung, and to hold onto anguish easily because the body is always waiting for more air. It's always in a state of anxiety. Shallow breathing keeps more waste circulating in the body, thereby using up extra B-complex nutrients. A depletion of B-complex compromises the nervous system.

Deep breathers inhale quantities of air that fill the lungs and push more oxygen into the blood. Consequently, they tend to be more relaxed and better able to adjust to life's ups-and-downs.

A person who plays the flute, sings, or practices yoga or martial arts, all of which utilize deep-breathing techniques, is better able to cleanse the body of waste. Good cells love oxygen. Diseased and dying cells do not, because oxygen causes them to die sooner. Diseased cells are free to continue swimming around and will stay in the body as microscopic corpses when they die off. They simply keep floating around in your system. But by breathing more deeply, you will eliminate more thoroughly and completely and not allow these dead cells to hang around to clog up your arteries, your joints, or your bowels. This is also another reason for exercise – it forces us to breathe in and out more deeply.

Here is a breathing exercise to try:

~ Exhale fully by forcing all the air out of your lungs.

~ Your next response will be to breathe in deeply and fully, which is good!

~ Repeat this exercise once every 30 minutes, or at least every hour.

Since you are expelling more of the waste material that disease, germs, and viruses use as food, you will be less likely to become sick. If the food for the disease is not present, the disease will not stay. If you don't feed it, it will not grow.

Look online for books and CDs about breath work.

It is not just the foods you take into your body that are important, but the liquids as well. Some health practitioners feel that putting food and liquid together dilutes the digestive juices. They recommend you drink any liquids either before or after meals. When you fully and completely chew your food, you should have enough saliva in your mouth to moisturize the food sufficiently so that swallowing is comfortable and easy.

Water

It used to be clean and it used to be free. Well, it's not free anymore, and tap water is not what I call clean. Somehow, we are always paying for water. There are myriad bottled waters on the market now, but not all are created equal. Most waters are sold in a plastic container, which is unfortunate. When left in sunlight or warmed in a microwave most plastics impart micro-particles into our food and drink. When a "dark field test" is administered to blood, many people exhibit the presence of polypropylene (a byproduct of some soft plastics) in their bloodstream. If you are aware and careful about this and do not leave containers in your car, the sun, or use plastic to cook or heat foods in the microwave, you will be fine.

I recommend 2 waters that are alkalizing: Fiji™ brand water, with a pH of 7.5, and gold label Trinity™ water (with a pH of 9.2). Trinity™ supplies two kinds of water, so read the labels carefully.

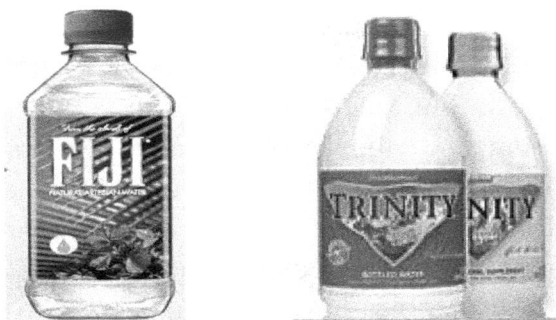

The general rule for full hydration is to drink daily *in ounces* a number equal to half your body weight. This means if you weigh 150 lbs, drink 75 ounces of good water. Most of us do not drink enough H2O.

Symptoms of dehydration include mental confusion and dementia. A lack of hydration may be implicated in Alzheimer's disease. Health practitioners find that simply hydrating a patient can reduce symptoms of senility and dementia.

Other symptoms of dehydration are acid indigestion and allergies. I like to think of it this way: A well-hydrated cell contains clean fluid, and is floating in clean fluid. An insufficiently hydrated cell is like a mud puddle; the cell floats in muddy water. Now, where do you want muddy puddles – in your brain? Your toenails? Your tongue? Your ears? I personally don't want *any* mud puddles!

If you drink half your body weight in ounces of water on a daily basis, you will be hydrated. Also keep in mind that you are cleaning your cells and flushing debris out of your body. There is a fine line, however, between enough and too much. Taking in too much water will flood your system and flush out precious nutrients.

One of the tests I like to show people is: Pinch the skin on the back of your hand. If the skin stays up and does not snap back fairly quickly, you are probably dehydrated and need more fluid. If the skin returns to normal fairly quickly, you are well-hydrated.

If you are drinking so much water that you must urinate every 5 minutes, that is excessive and you are probably losing nutrition and not waste material. Seek a happy medium by using common sense.

Some of you are wondering about using distilled water. Distilled water is *empty* water, and empty water goes into your body looking to be filled up. Plain, distilled water drunk on a regular basis will deplete your body of nutrition. If you need to use distilled water, doctor it up with a generous pinch of gray sea salt for each gallon of water. After all, our body fluid is a lot closer to ocean water than anything else. It won't taste salty, I promise! It will, however, contain elements that assist your cellular structure to hydrate and bathe without robbing them of nutrients. Sometimes I take it a step further by adding 1 teaspoon to 1 tablespoon of a liquid antioxidant (like chlorophyll, mangosteen, Goji™, or Noni™ juice) or a multivitamin/multimineral (again, in liquid form) along with sea salt.

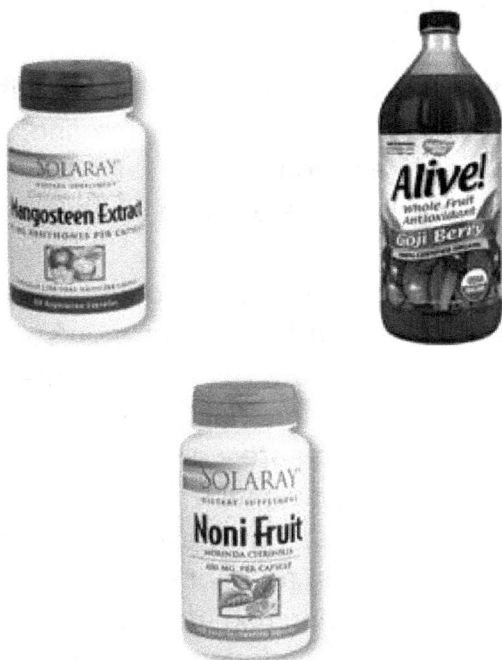

Noni has been used by Polynesian cultures for over 1500 years. It is very helpful for degenerative diseases and provides anti-tumor and anti-inflammatory effects. An alternative is pomegranate juice, which tastes great and is easier to find. Pomegranate juice may also cost less.

The Little Book of Self-Health

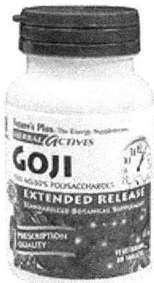

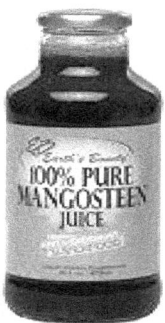

Antioxidants, which are also anti-aging, are high in vitamins E and C. They help protect against heart disease, cancer, and chronic degenerative diseases. Combinations of antioxidants provide protection against free radicals, molecules that bind to healthy cells and create damage. We all need and have a small quantity of free radicals in our bodies for the elimination of diseased and dying cells. But having too many free radicals destroys healthy cells.

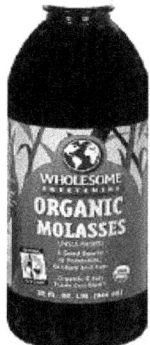

Rich in minerals and vitamins, unsulphured molasses has more calcium than milk, more iron than eggs, and more potassium than any other food. Our great-grandmothers used it as a tonic, with 1 teaspoon or tablespoon of molasses to 4-8 ounces of warm water. Organic is not required but do choose unsulphured blackstrap molasses.

7
CLEANSING, FASTING, COLONICS

We live in a society and culture that is literally contaminated with toxins and pollutants that are harmful to our bodies. Consequently, we need to take measures to cleanse the body periodically to remove all these harmful toxins. Remember that when toxins remain in the body, bad bacteria will ferment and leech into and contaminate surrounding organs, setting up cells to accept disease. This will also cross-contaminate other internal functions, producing a wide variety of symptoms and ailments. Seasonal cleansing is worth consideration.

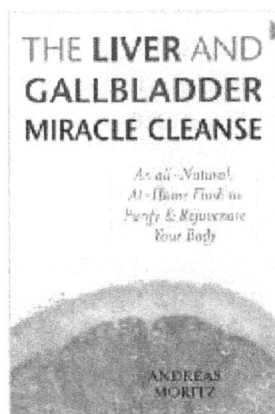

THE **LIVER** AND
GALLBLADDER
MIRACLE CLEANSE

An all-Natural,
At-Home Flush to
Purify & Rejuvenate
Your Body

ANDREAS
MORITZ

"The Liver and Gallbladder Miracle Cleanse" book by Andreas Moritz is the best written, with complete explanations of how, why, and when to cleanse. It contains so much for you to learn! You will find it easy to follow.

Cleansing from mouth to anus once or twice a year is not only a good idea, one should consider it a requirement. If you have emerging symptoms or are dealing with an ongoing illness, you may need to cleanse your digestive system even more than twice a year.

Colonics

This could mean a series of enemas or "high colonics." High colonics are a complete intestinal and colon wash. The procedure takes about an hour and is performed in a clinical setting. A practitioner uses disposable equipment to push water in rectally (up from the bottom), which allows toxins and fecal matter to drain out.

Herbal Cleanses

Your local health food store or vitamin shop can help you select any one of a number of available cleansing programs, including herbal cleanses you can use at home (previously mentioned). These might be in pill form or as a powder to mix with juice. If you choose a 30-day cleanse, keep in mind that you may experience flu-like symptoms, rashes, and/or headaches. Or, all your body's orifices may discharge at one time, which is a good sign! This may just be your body's way of expunging toxins. These symptoms will decrease in proportion and dissipate as toxin levels decrease and your system begins to flow freely. Such symptoms might occur at any time as you clean up your internal organs. The body has to gather useless material and toxins, banishing them via the closest exit.

Fasting

You can fast 1 day a week for 3 days, or for 10 consecutive days. Before fasting, research fasting "recipes" and read all you can about them. I don't recommend a water fast unless you have already fasted for 3 or 10 days with juices or teas.

Food, water, oxygen, and the toilet. Eat, drink, breathe, poop, and you will be merry! I tell people that every cell in our bodies must eat, drink, breathe, go potty, and have fun. If one or more of these is missing, cells will break down, leading to disease.

Be patient with yourself. If the oldest cell in your body is 7 years old, it literally could take up to 7 years to rid yourself of a specific symptom or ailment because that is how long it takes the body to regenerate its oldest cells. It takes 9 months to "build" a baby, which is, at its foundation, cell construction. We must remove damaged and diseased cells so that new cells will have a home. This can take some time, even if you are using only natural products. If you take unnatural or manmade products, your body will then have to deal with the contaminants and alien components, which may prolong the healing process.

Some chemistries, like pharmaceutical medicines prescribed by medical doctors, provide your brain a signal that says, "Oh, you don't have that symptom anymore, so you must be feeling better." This doesn't mean that the ailment or illness is actually gone; it just means that the symptoms have been *treated* (as opposed to *cured*), so that a chemical reaction signals the brain that you no longer have that problem. When this occurs, the only choice the ailment has is to get your attention by growing worse in another part of the body. This is so you will know that there is still a condition needing to be healed. As a naturopath and a health & healing advocate, I like to work on the underlying condition while helping clients deal with their symptoms.

Educate yourself thoroughly before fasting. There are a number of books for guidance on this.

Lotions

We apply a variety of lotions, oils, perfumes, shampoos, and cosmetics all over our bodies. These products are absorbed through the skin and into our system. Since our bodies are already fighting pollutants, toxins, and chemicals, why apply even more chemistry to our skins?

Skin is an organ of elimination of toxins and waste products. Therefore, the rule for products that go on the body is the same as for products that go *in* the body – high-quality natural and organic products are best. Using low-quality chemical products is like poisoning your system. Natural products exist, so use them! Don't be fooled by commercials and labels that say, "all natural." As with food, if the ingredients are unrecognizable, they probably aren't good for you.

Follow your "gut feelings" as they go hand-in-hand with common sense.

If pure products are too expensive, use emu oil, mink oil, coconut, or olive oil added to aloe. Add lavender or tea tree oil for their healing properties, or pure essential oils for fragrance or aromatherapy. I call it kitchen chemistry and I always say, if I wouldn't eat this product, why assimilate it through my skin?

> **The difference between a successful person and others is not a lack of strength, not a lack of knowledge, but rather a lack of will.**
> **Anonymous**

The Little Book of Self-Health

8
WEIGHT LOSS – WEIGHT GAIN

As your body gets the proper nutrients, your cravings will diminish, as will those times you put food into your mouth without thinking. When the body is satisfied nutritionally, it won't signal that it wants food. If your nutritional foundation is not solid, your brain will keep telling you that you are hungry.

There is a biochemical process that creates hunger and the cravings that lead to weight gain. It occurs when the body thinks it will die from starvation. To find out how this works, read on.

When you use this program over time, your body will find its natural weight. That may be heavier than you are currently (or than you picture your ideal self) or it may be lighter. The body knows what weight it should be, and when it has the nutrients it needs, it will stay at approximately that weight, usually within 5 pounds or so. When the proper nutrient level is reached, the body naturally turns off the hunger signals until sufficient calories have been burned. Hunger arises when the body needs more *nutrients*, not simply more calories.

With this program, your taste for foods will change too. You will begin to notice that some foods don't taste as good as they used to. You will also notice that other foods you previously disliked now appeal to you. Some of my clients have reported developing the ability to taste, smell, and feel the chemicals and waxes in packaged, processed, and fast foods. But they like this new ability! It helps them to help themselves.

Starvation, crash diets, and most fad diets do not create the necessary nutritional foundation for safe, healthy, and sustainable weight loss. If the nutritional foundation is not satisfied there will always be a feeling of "never enough." It could take 2½ to 3 months before your emotional body is willing to let go of excess, as over that time period the feeling of "not getting enough" fades away.

Immune-Building Products

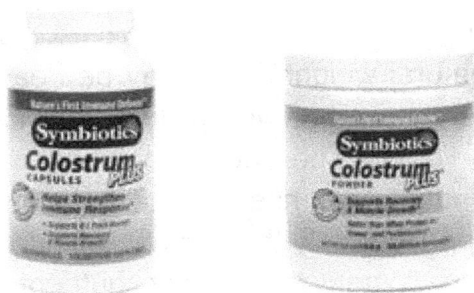

Colostrum is one of the best immune-building products on the market. Not the cheapest, but one of the best. All colostrums are good or even great. Pick a brand that suits your budget.

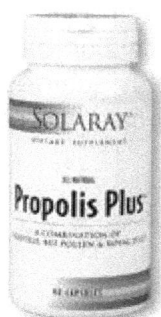

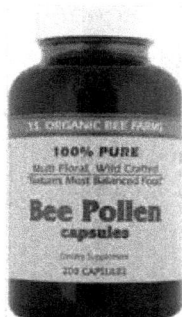

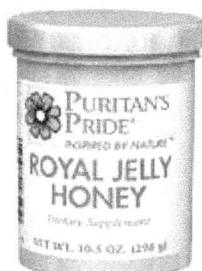

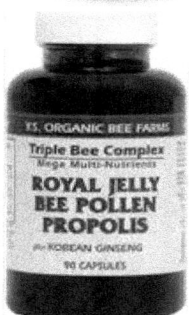

I call these the "3 Bees." Together they comprise a virtually complete multi-vitamin/multimineral. Anti-aging and antioxidant benefits, too. Also available combined as shown.

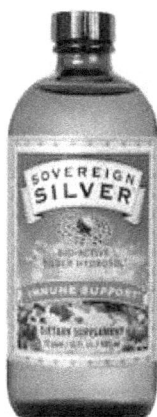

Ultra-fine silver solution contains smaller particles than colloidal silver. Both are universally used as natural antibiotics. The product proves toxic to most fungi, bacteria (including anthrax), parasites, and many viruses. Not for use by pregnant or nursing women. The ultra fine silver solution will not turn skin blue or gray. There are also several brands of machines for making your own silver products. You can find out more through research online.

9
MASSAGE

In addition to my nutritional work and research, I teach massage arts to students working toward certification, and have a massage practice of many years.

Massage was the first *hands-on* healing art. For thousands of years, people receiving massage have found new mobility and range of motion for their sore, stiff muscles. These improvements apply to tendons and ligaments too. Therapeutic massage creates positive changes in the cellular structure and soft tissues of the whole body. It is both *passive exercise* and *preventive medicine* by creating a comfortable feeling throughout the mind, body, and spirit.

Massage is a great way to nurture and calm the nerves, increase blood flow, and clear toxins while relaxing sore muscles. Light or deep tissue massage therapy can transform any stiff, sore, aching body into a soft, supple, flexible unit. Massage also promotes relaxation by reducing stress and stimulating the body's own ability to help itself heal, all the while helping to ease blocked emotional and physical trauma. With massage, you'll feel more energy and better focus because it increases blood flow to the brain. Nothing can replace a great massage! It is not an indulgence, but rather an effective tool for healing.

The best massage therapists are caring, compas-
sionate people helping others feel great in their physical, mental, and spiritual bodies.

HUGS
Hugging is healthy.
It helps the body's immune system;
it keeps you healthier, it cures depression,
it reduces stress,
it induces sleep, it's invigorating and rejuvenating.
It has no unpleasant side effects.
Hugging is no less than a miracle drug.
Hugging is all-natural; it is organic, naturally sweet,
contains no pesticides, no preservatives, no
artificial ingredients,
and is 100% wholesome.
Hugging is practically perfect;
with no removable parts, no batteries to wear out,
no periodic check-ups and low energy
consumption,
high energy yield, inflation-proof, non-fattening,
no monthly payments, no insurance requirements,
theft-proof, non-taxable, non-polluting,
and of course, fully returnable.
Author Unknown

Dosage
   4 hugs per day for survival
   8 hugs per day for maintenance
   12 hugs per day for growth

The healing value of touch through massage or
hugging cannot be quantified. Healthy connection with

other beings is a vital and important part of being human, and is therefore an important component to health and balance. I highly recommend it.

Lymphatic Clearing

A one-hour lymph-clearing session uses state-of-the-art vibrational medicine and massage techniques.

In Greek, "lymph" means "a pure, clear stream." A single lymphatic system numbers close to one trillion cells. It works hand-in-hand with the immune and blood systems by collecting toxins and waste from the entire body. Lymph nodes counteract infection by filtering the lymph fluid. They also customize antibodies to kill and remove bacteria and foreign substances. Lymph organs include bone marrow, the thymus gland, the spleen, tonsils, adenoids, lymph nodes, and appendix. If any of these organs are missing due to disease, dysfunction, or surgical removal, your lymph system is working overtime 24-hours a day.

Systems of a dysfunctional lymph system include allergies and food sensitivities, colds, influenza, joint pain, headaches, menstrual cramps, arthritis, fibrocystic breasts, sinusitis, loss of appetite, gastrointestinal challenges, muscle cramping, swollen tissue, fatigue, mental fuzziness, depression, parasites, acne, cellulite, and lymphoma and other cancers.

Lymph and blood systems are like heads and tails of the same coin. Whatever affects one affects the other. So, every cell of the body is affected to the good or bad.

10
EMOTIONAL & SPIRITUAL HEALTH

Fear, anger, shame, resentment, and guilt are responsible for more symptoms of ill health than any other influence. Which begs the question: Does your attitude help or hinder your physical body? I have discovered that mental attitude, often overlooked and discounted by most, plays a major role in our quest for a healthier lifestyle.

Everything in the human body is connected to the brain. Learning to keep the information highways and byways "in the moment" as much as possible will serve us well. Keep in mind that when you wake up tomorrow you have a whole new day to work on staying in the moment. When we project into the future, we don't deal with the NOW.

Drawing or imagining a healthy heart, lungs, or liver, tells your body what you want to have happen. Find pictures of healthy cells, a healthy colon, brain, etc., and tell your body that health is what you want. We don't have to tell the body how to achieve that goal, just like we don't have to tell it how to heal a paper cut. The body *knows* what to do. We must become aware of allowing our body's natural language to come through. The body talks to us all the time with what are called "symptoms," or "feelings and impressions."

When we say things like, "My bad hip is giving me trouble today," our brain thinks "bad hip" and makes it happen: "Oh, you want a bad hip...well, here it is! Call me bad and I will be just that."

Thoughts are physical actions; they move brain cells. Those actions, reactions, and interactions have force and an outcome – positive or negative – which in turn moves other cells toward good or not so good. We have much greater control over ourselves than we might sometimes realize.

Remember when you were a child with a test to take at school? You told your mother you felt sick. The more convincing you had to be with Mom, the more you actually felt ill. But as soon as the bus left or Mom went off to work, you felt better!

Tell your body what you want *from* it and *for* it, then tell it the things you are doing to help it reach that goal. At the very least, you will laugh while talking to your liver, bowel, hip, or knee. Laughter helps the healing process!

Guided Imagery/Hypnosis

Both guided imagery and hypnosis put the conscious mind and subconscious mind on the same page. The whole body is affected by what happens in the mind.

Our subconscious can help or hurt the healing process and affect how effectively our cellular body is functioning. When you learn to help your mind help itself, every part of your life will improve. Guided imagery and hypnosis can give you the tools and exercises to accomplish this.

We are the most evolved beings on the planet and have the ability to change our minds. You can learn to change your mind for daily positive results!

Look in your area for a qualified practitioner. Trust is involved so take your time finding the right person.

> **When the day is over and you have done your best, wait the results in peace.**
> **Anonymous**

11
SUMMARY & CLOSING

We must be willing to experiment. Human bodies are like snowflakes – no two are alike. You will need to be patient and diligent. The cleaner your internal body, the better your health. The more natural, organic nutrients absorbed and assimilated by the body, the faster they body will heal and the sooner you will feel how great it is to be alive and well.

You are maintaining a healthy lifestyle when you eat healthy food and incorporate food nutrients in the form of liquid vitamins and green drinks. Be sure to include a periodic cleansing in conjunction with exercise and spiritual practice, or mental health/stress reduction practices. Then, if you should encounter a surge of pollutants or toxins, or eat unhealthy foods, your body will be better able to fight off the effects and more quickly and efficiently rid your system of their potential damage. No-one knows exactly how healthy a particular body can be, because in no person have all cells reproduced with more health than the previous generation of cells. Imagine if such a healthy scenario were to take place!

I hope through this book you have learned how the human body works and what it needs for optimal health. You need not take my word on the subjects explained herein – check each and every detail for yourself. You'll learn what works for you and what doesn't, plus a whole lot more.

I wish you a full and healthy life!

> **To a wise man, every day is a new life.**
> **Anonymous**

THIS YEAR

Write a love letter. Share some treasure.
Mend a quarrel. Seek out a forgotten friend.
Dismiss a suspicion and replace it with trust.
Give a soft answer. Encourage a youth.
Manifest your loyalty in word and deed.
Keep a promise. Find the time. Forego a grudge.
Forgive an enemy.
LISTEN…
Apologize if you are wrong.
Try to understand. Rout envy.
Examine your demands on others.
Think first of someone else.
Appreciate. Be kind. Be gentle. Laugh a little.
Laugh a little more.
Deserve confidence. Take up arms
against malice.
Decry complacency. Express your gratitude.
HAVE FAITH…
Welcome a stranger. Gladden the heart
of a child.
Take pleasure in the beauty and wonder
of the earth.
SPEAK YOUR LOVE.
SPEAK IT AGAIN.
Then…
SPEAK IT ONCE AGAIN…

Author Unknown

RECOMMENDED READING

Healthy Healing: A Guide to Self-Healing for Everyone, by Linda Rector Page, N.D., Ph.D.

Prescription for Nutritional Healing: A Practical A-Z Reference to Drug-Free Remedies Using Vitamins, Minerals, Herbs and Food Supplements, by James F. Balch, MD, and Phyllis A. Balch, C.N.C.

Spontaneous Healing, by Andrew Weil, MD (and any other book by Dr. Weil)

Ten Essential Herbs, by Lalitha Thomas

Herbs of Grace, and, *Becoming Independently Healthy,* by Farida Sharan

School of Natural Healing, by John R. Christopher, N.D., Master Herbalist

The Liver and Gallbladder Miracle Cleanse, by Andreas Moritz

Anti-Aging Manual: The Encyclopedia of Natural Health, by Joseph B. Marion

ABOUT THE AUTHOR

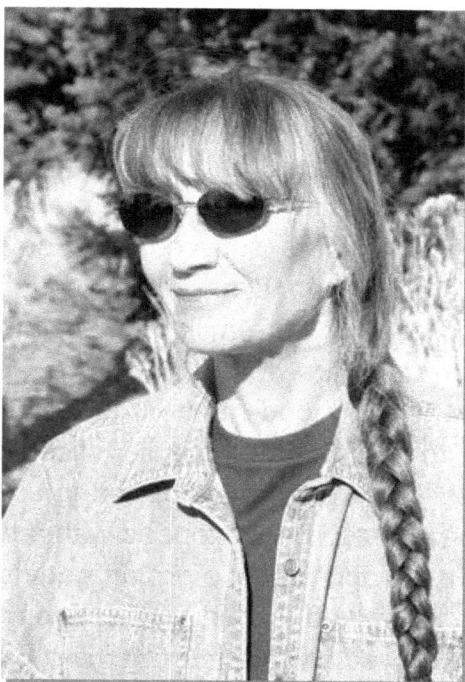

Toni Fain holds a Doctor of Natural Medicine from Arkansas College of Natural Health (formerly Southern College of Naturopathy). Her 40+ years of study and practice include two years' study of Native American medicine in Flagstaff, Arizona, and two years studying with a Chinese apothecary (pharmacist) in Oakland, California.

Dr. Fain now makes her home in Nevada. For many years she taught the art of massage therapy to students seeking licensure. In addition to her own health and healing practice, she provides continuing education instruction for massage therapists.

Fain's first encounters with natural healing came during her early years at her grandparent's home, where she gathered garden herbs and vegetables for the "anti-gas" tea offered after large holiday meals. There were plenty of fresh vegetable soups, and healing teas whenever the children fell ill. Grandmother made what she called gravy, made from a blend of veggies thinned with either some pan juice or tomato juice. Fain's brothers suffered from severe allergies and ear problems, and her father suffered with indigestion. The three were milk drinkers while symptom-free family members were not.

One early childhood memory is of her grandmother's cure for a cold: fresh garlic, sliced onions, sage leaves, and rosemary, all wrapped in a dishtowel laid across the afflicted chest, topped with a heating pad.

Fain's massage practice got an early start when as a child she walked on her father's back (as a firefighter he carried people from burning buildings). She later graduated to using elbows, fists, and thumbs to loosen cranky muscles and in her teens practiced massage within her mother's hair salon.

She employed natural healing techniques with her own children and has not consulted a medical doctor since her youngest child's birth in 1981. Now in her late 50s, Fain takes no prescription or OTC drugs. She works 40+ hours a week.

Though she indulges occasionally in fast food (no cheese!) and rich desserts (even for breakfast), she is also known to carry small packs of sea salt, fresh rosemary, thyme, cinnamon, and/or B-grade maple syrup when eating out. She's quick to explain, "It's not about perfection, it's about finding a balance" through countering negative health habits with positive choices. Her personal goal – REgeneration instead of DEgeneration.

This book was originally published in 1997 under the title "Life is for Living." That original derived from numerous studies and practices by Toni Fain, whose pursuit of a deep and abiding foundation for natural healing and health took her to Mexico, Moscow (in the USSR), Berkeley, Utah, Arkansas, and Arizona. In this expanded version she adds even more insight and instruction.

INDEX

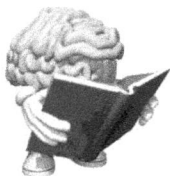

This is your brain absorbing helpful information about your body and good nutrition.

Published by Toni Fain Healing Arts
Author photo – Paula Riley
Brain illustration – Clipart.com
Text set in Arial font